I0421028

Asthma Treatment 101

Diet, Cure, and Natural Remedies to be Asthma-free Naturally

© **Copyright 2014 by SIASA Ventures - All rights reserved.**

This document is geared towards providing exact and reliable information with regards to the topic and issue covered. The publication is sold with the idea that the publisher is not required to render accounting, officially permitted, or otherwise, qualified services. If advice is necessary, legal or professional, a practiced individual in the profession should be ordered.

- From a Declaration of Principles which was accepted and approved equally by a Committee of the American Bar Association and a Committee of Publishers and Associations.

In no way is it legal to reproduce, duplicate, or transmit any part of this document in either electronic means or in printed format. Recording of this publication is strictly prohibited and any storage of this document is not allowed unless with written permission from the publisher. All rights reserved.

The information provided herein is stated to be truthful and consistent, in that any liability, in terms of inattention or otherwise, by any usage or abuse of any policies, processes, or directions contained within is the solitary and utter responsibility of the recipient reader. Under no circumstances will any legal responsibility or blame be held against the publisher for any reparation, damages, or monetary loss due to the information herein, either directly or indirectly.

Respective authors own all copyrights not held by the publisher.

The information herein is offered for informational purposes solely, and is universal as so. The presentation of the information is without contract or any type of guarantee assurance.

The trademarks that are used are without any consent, and the publication of the trademark is without permission or backing by the trademark owner. All trademarks and brands within this book are for clarifying purposes only and are the owned by the owners themselves, not affiliated with this document.

Table of Contents

Introduction

I want to thank you and congratulate you for downloading the book, *"Asthma Treatment 101"*.

This book contains a basic background on asthma—how it happens and its categories. In addition, it also contains proven steps and strategies that could effectively manage asthma and keep it under control for the rest of your life.

Asthma can affect how you live your life. It limits the things you can do. You spend lots of sick days because of it.

Even when your symptoms are mild, you can't perform at your top potential because of fatigue. Worse, you get anxious about having an attack.

This book will show that although incurable, the symptoms of asthma can be controlled. Several medications and remedies are available to manage the symptoms of your condition, allowing you to live a comfortable and normal life.

Learn all you have to know to fully understand and take control of this condition. Read on, transform your life, and be asthma-free.

Thanks again for downloading this book, I hope you will enjoy it!

CHAPTER 1
Asthma at a Glance

Asthma is a chronic respiratory illness defined primarily by airway obstruction, which responds spontaneously and with treatment.

Inflammation, as a result of over-reactive airways, is the main culprit of the said obstruction. The occurrence of this disease is attributed to an interplay between genetics and environmental factors.

During an asthma attack, the airways become inflamed and swollen, which make the respiratory tract extraordinarily sensitive to irritants.

This allows the entire respiratory system to become susceptible to allergic reactions. Exposure to substances that normally do not trigger allergic reactions now initiates asthmatic symptoms.

The airways become constricted because of the cumulative effects of swollen air passages and increased mucus production.

Airflow throughout the lungs becomes severely restricted. Less oxygen enters the body, consequently leading to the accumulation of carbon dioxide within the blood and tissues.

One of the distinguishing features of asthma as opposed to other respiratory conditions is the timing of the occurrence of its symptoms—it is often worse at night and during the early hours of the morning.

Although asthma is considered an incurable condition, it can be effectively managed and kept under control with the right management and treatment plan.

HISTORY OF ASTHMA

Although a connotation of respiratory distress was first used in China way back 2600 BC, it was Hippocrates who first coined the term "Asthma", a Greek word meaning "wind" or "blow" to describe panting or respiratory distress.

He was also the first physician who associated respiratory distress with the environment. Hence, he was considered by some as the first "allergist".

At around 50AD, Pliny the Elder noticed that pollens actually caused respiratory distress and recommended that ephedra from red wine should be used as a remedy.

Several improvements occurred after then, but it was not until the 1900s when immunotherapy was introduced as a treatment modality for asthma.

During the 20th century, different medicines such as epinephrine, aminophylline and isoprotenerol were used to treat asthma.

In 1969, doctors began to use inhaled bronchodilators to treat asthma as these were found to have less adverse effects on the heart and were available for short term and long-term use.

Inhaled corticosteroids also had less systemic side effects as opposed to oral medications.

Despite the fact that asthma has been discovered for over millions of years, over 25 million people in the United States alone still suffer from this condition.

This only shows that there is so much more to discover about this disease.

DEMOGRAPHICS AND DISEASE PREVALENCE

Asthma is a chronic disease that affects the respiratory tract. Almost 300 million people across the world are affected by this condition. 15% of children and 10 to 12% of adults have been diagnosed with asthma.

That being said, asthma is truly among the most relevant diseases that must be paid close attention to.

In developing countries, the prevalence of asthma is said to be increasing. This increase is attributed to over-urbanization.

The conditions of these individuals are mostly related to atopy. Allergens like dust mites and other pollutants play a high role.

During childhood stages, studies have found that males are twice as likely to get asthma than females. However, as they reach adulthood, the ratio begins to equalize.

WHAT HAPPENS DURING AN ASTHMA ATTACK

An asthma attack begins with an exposure to a trigger. When this happens, the smooth muscles surrounding the air passages start to swell and constrict.

Airflow is restricted. Inflammation in the respiratory tract worsens, causing further narrowing of the air passages.

Aside from bronchoconstriction, airway obstruction is also attributed to edema, vascular congestion and luminal occlusion with exudates. Because of these, oxygen levels in the blood and tissues drop.

In order to compensate for the hypoxic condition, the lungs act by increasing breathing rate in an attempt to improve oxygen availability. The increased demand on the lungs worsens inflammation.

As inflammation worsens, the lungs and the rest of the respiratory tract produce more mucus in order to protect its tissues from damage.

This, in fact, is a vicious cycle that can worsen and turn fatal if adequate and prompt management is not given.

Persons suffering from an asthma stack may manifest with clammy and bluish skin.

They usually prefer to sit with elbow in the knees, and may even prefer sitting than lying down. They also have difficulty speaking.

TYPES

There are different types of asthma, depending on the triggers and age of onset.

Child-onset

This type of asthma starts during the childhood years. It often begins when a child is exposed to common allergens and becomes sensitized to these. Genetics play a huge role in this.

Atopic conditions increase the risk for developing child-onset asthma. This is a genetically influenced hypersensitivity state to common environmental allergens.

Children suffering from asthma are often hospitalized, thus causing school absenteeism.

Among the most common causes of asthma in children are exercise (>80%0, infections (bronchitis, flu), allergy, drugs, irritants, weather, chemicals, pets and emotions.

Adult-onset

This refers to asthma that develops when a person is already more than 20 years old. This condition is more common among women.

Adult-onset asthma is also less common compared to the child-onset type.

Often, this type is triggered by exposure to certain allergic materials or by the presence of other forms of allergies.

Exercise-induced

Coughing, wheezing or feeling out of breath during exercise or afterwards is an indication of exercise-induced asthma.

It is normal to feel winded, especially if starting out on an exercise routine.

However, if the coughing and breathing difficulties are worse than usual or when not in proportion with the intensity of exercise, then it could be asthma.

Exercise-induced asthma occurs more commonly in people living in cold regions.

Cough-induced

This is one of the most difficult types of asthma to diagnose. The symptoms overlap with those of cough.

The doctor would have to eliminate the presence of other possible problems such as sinus diseases, chronic bronchitis, and post-nasal drip (from hay fever).

It may take a long time and a few repeated episodes before a concrete diagnosis can be made.

Occupational Asthma

Asthma symptoms triggered by exposure to chemicals and substances in the workplace is classified as occupational asthma. Common triggers include gases, vapors, dust, smoke, fumes, and chemicals.

It may also be due to exposure to animal products, humidity, pollen, temperature, molds, and viruses.

This type often manifests when a person starts a new job and ends when leaving that particular job.

If the trigger is removed within 6 months after the initial exposure, complete recovery may ensue. Otherwise, irreversible airway changes may already take place.

Nocturnal asthma

The symptoms manifest between the hours of midnight and 8 in the morning. These are often due to exposure to allergens present in the home such as pet dander or dust.

It may also be due to sinus conditions. Sometimes, people who suffer from this type of asthma do not experience any symptoms during the day.

They often experience wheezing when lying down.

Symptoms also become worse around 2 to 4 in the morning.

This can be attributed to the following factors: gastric reflux, sleeping position, and drop of cortisone and epinephrine levels at night.

Severe asthma (steroid-resistant type)

Most asthma conditions are effectively managed with the administration of steroid medications.

In some people, asthma symptoms become more troublesome. Steroids are the usual medications used in treating asthma. They act by relaxing the airways and inhibiting mucus production.

However, in some instances, the condition declines but no longer improves with steroid medications.

This may be due to prolonged use of the said medications or may be due to the gradual worsening of asthma over a period of years.

In these cases, more aggressive treatment methods may already be required in order to effectively control asthma attacks.

RISK FACTORS

Several factors are linked to increased risks of developing asthma conditions, including:

- Presence of allergic conditions
  - Atopy is the major risk factor of asthma. Patients with asthma almost always suffer from other conditions such as allergic rhinitis and allergic dermatitis (eczema). However, in developing countries, not all patients with history of atopy become asthmatic. This stresses the impact of environmental factors.
- Airway hyperresponsiveness
  - This is the physiologic abnormality of asthmatic patients, characterized by excessive bronchoconstrictive response to allergens, which would not have any effect on normal airways.
- Genetic predisposition (family history of asthma)
  - The severity of asthma is said to be genetically determined.

- Diet
  - Deficiency in Vitamin D may predispose to asthma. In addition, the following food may trigger asthma: food containing benzoates and sulphite, foods containing yeast or mold, foods containing coloring, some dairy products and nuts.
- Smoking
  - Smoking asthmatics have more severe conditions and are hospitalized more frequently
- Obesity
  - Obesity is an independent risk factor for asthma, particularly in women.
- Exposure to second-hand smoke
- In-utero exposure to cigarettes (i.e. pregnant mothers who smoke or pregnant mothers exposed to second-hand smoke)
- Exposure to triggers in the workplace (i.e. chemicals in farming, hairdressing, manufacturing plants, etc.)
- Other risk factors: maternal age, duration of breastfeeding, prematurity, low birth weight and inactivity

CHAPTER 2

Causes and Symptoms

Asthma symptoms are triggered after exposure to allergens and other triggers. As the body becomes sensitized, it exhibits hypersensitivity reactions.

COMMON TRIGGERS

Common triggers include the following:

- Allergens
  - Allergens activate inflammatory cells in the body, which results to a cascade of steps leading to bronchoconstriction. *Dermatophagoides* are the most common allergens that trigger asthma. Other allergens include pet dander, cockroaches, pollens and spores.
- Smoke, such as from tobacco and burning leaves and wood
- Air pollution
  - Increased levels of noxious fumes, sulfur dioxide, nitrogen oxide and ozone are associated with asthma attacks.
- Stress
  - Stress and psychological factors induce asthma attack via the cholinergic reflex pathway.
- Infections
  - Respiratory Syncytial Virus has been associated with the development of asthma in infancy, although the pathogenesis is yet to be elucidated.
- Food
  - Several patients have claimed that they experienced asthma attack after consuming particular kinds of food.

However, the pathogenesis of this is yet to be elucidated. Metabisulfite, a food preservative, releases sulfur dioxide gas in the stomach, triggering asthma. Tartrazine, a yellow food coloring, is also said to be an asthma trigger.

- Some pharmacologic agents (drugs)
  - o Beta-adrenergic agents commonly trigger asthma. Hence, asthmatic patients should avoid these drugs since they cause bronchoconstriction. Angiotensin-converting enzyme inhibitors (ACE-Inhibitors) theoretically cause asthma attacks, but they rarely happen in reality. Aspirin may also be detrimental to asthmatic patients.

- Exercise
  - o Exercise is a common trigger of asthma in children, as it indirectly activates inflammatory cells, leading to bronchoconstriction. Exercise-induced asthma usually occurs at the end of exercise and resolves spontaneously after approximately 30 minutes. This condition occurs more frequently in cold countries. Hence, athletes in these regions are advised to use inhaled corticosteroids regularly, especially before sports activities.

- Physical factors
  - o Cold air and hyperventilation are also causes of asthma attack. In addition, laughter is also a common trigger. Although the mechanism is still uncertain, strong smells are also said to be triggers of asthma attack.

- Hormonal factors
  - o Some women have severe asthma attacks before their menses. This is related to the drop of progesterone levels. Hence, treatment with oral progesterone may help. Hormonal factors are also seen in patients with thyrotoxicosis and hypothyroidism, which are also related to asthma attacks.

- Gastroesophageal Reflux
  - o Gastroesophageal reflux occurs as a result of chronic use of bronchodilators. However, asthmatic patients

taking anti-reflux therapy are still not spared by attacks.

SYMPTOMS

Asthmatic patients typically present with wheezing (high-pitched sound that is heard during exhalation), dyspnea and coughing.

Symptoms generally range from mild respiratory difficulties to severe respiratory distress. These symptoms may appear at various intervals and frequencies, depending on the triggering factors and overall health. There are some people who experience asthma symptoms on a consistent basis.

During an asthma attack, symptoms include:

- Pain or tightness felt over the chest area
- Shortness of breath
- Wheezing or whistling sounds when breathing out – wheezing is a symptom common among children who suffer from asthma
- Difficulty sleeping because of wheezing, coughing, or shortness of breath
- Wheezing or coughing episodes worsened by the presence of respiratory viruses, such as those that cause flu or colds
- Night cough, since asthma is worse at night

Signs that indicate worsening asthma conditions include:

- Asthma attacks become more frequent, with symptoms becoming more severe
- Breathing increasingly becomes more difficult, which can be measured by a peak flow meter (a device that measures how well the lungs are functioning)
- Increasing need to use inhalers for quick-relief

In some individuals, asthma symptoms worsen in certain instances such as:

- Exposure to dry and cold air, which is more frequently seen in people who suffer from exercise-induced type of asthma

- Exposure to irritants in the workplace such as gases, dust, and chemical fumes (these are commonly associated with occupational asthma)
- Exposure to allergens like those found in pollen, cockroaches, and pet dander (common among people who suffer from allergy-induced asthma)

Asthma symptoms can worsen rapidly, over the course of a few minutes to hours. It is important to provide treatment and relief measures as soon as asthma attack starts.

Diagnosis of Asthma

The following tests are usually requested when an individual presents with symptoms of asthma:

- Pulmonary Function Tests
  - Factors the affect the Pulmonary Function Tests (PFTs) include age, height, ethnicity and sex. Normal values include those >85%.
- Spirometry Test
  - This is the most frequently performed test to determine lung function. This test involves the use of a spirometer, a device used to measure the amount of air one can hold, and one's ability to move air in and out of the lungs.
- Chest x-ray
  - Patients with severe asthma present with hyper-inflated lungs. During acute attack, pneumothorax (air inside the lungs) may ensue.
- Blood Gas Analysis
  - This indicates the status of blood gas exchange. This serves as the basis of the amount of oxygen to be given to the patient.
- Other hematologic tests
  - Total serum levels of IgE and IgE levels in relation to certain allergens may be measured. However, this test has not proven to be very useful in the diagnosis of asthma.

- Exhaled Nitric oxide
  - This is a non-invasive test to measure eosinophilic airway inflammation. This can also be used as a test to measure the patient's compliance to medications since the asthmatic patient's usual elevated levels may be suppressed by inhaled corticosteroid therapy.

Seeking emergency treatment

Severe attacks can be fatal, especially if not managed properly and promptly. Signs that a person suffering from attack needs emergency care include:

- No improvement in the severity of current symptoms even after using quick-relief inhalers like albuterol
- Rapidly worsening wheezing or shortness of breath
- Experiencing shortness of breath even with minimal effort or physical activity

PROGNOSIS

Asthma rarely results to death. This is especially evident in developing countries. The decrease in mortality secondary to asthma has been attributed to the use of inhaled corticosteroids.

Risk factors of mortality due to asthma include poorly controlled disease with frequent use of bronchodilators, poor compliance to steroid therapy and history of frequent hospitalization due to asthma attack.

A condition called status asthmaticus occurs when an asthma attack no longer responds to bronchodilators, which may lead to symptoms of potential respiratory failure.

This is a life-threatening condition, which requires immediate medical attention. This may be brought about by poor control of allergens or asthma triggers at home or at the workplace.

These patients may have poor compliance to medications.

Symptoms of status asthmaticus may include persistent shortness of breath and inability to speak. To avoid hospitalization, begin immediate treatment at first signs of symptoms.

Oxygenation is the primary treatment modality in patients experiencing status asthmaticus. Other medications as prescribed by the physician should be given as well.

CHAPTER 3
Natural Treatments

The basic goal in the treatment of asthma is to reduce inflammation. The aim is to control symptoms and exacerbations and to limit emergency room visits.

MEDICATIONS FOR ASTHMA

The following treatment modalities are the most commonly used in treating asthma:

- Bronchodilators- act on the smooth muscles of the airways to relieve bronchoconstriction.
    - o B2 Adrenergic agonists- used to relax smooth muscle cells of the airways
    - o Anticholinergics- prevent bronchoconstriction and mucus production
    - o Theophylline- used as an additional bronchodilator in patients with severe asthma
- Controller therapies- include inhaled steroids, which are the most commonly used controllers for asthma
    - o Inhaled corticosteroids- most effective controller for asthma
    - o Systemic corticosteroids- used intravenously to control severe asthma
    - o Antileukotrienes- less effective than inhaled corticosteroids but are useful add-ons for patients who do not respond well to low doses of inhaled corticosteroids
    - o Cromones- useful in treating exercise-induced asthma since they block sensory nerve activation

- Steroid-sparing therapies- include methotrexate, cyclosporin A, azathioprine, gold and IV gamma globulin. These groups of medications have not been proven to have long-term benefits. In addition, they also carry with them a long list of side effects.
- Anti-IgE- this treatment is expensive, but has been shown to reduce the number of exacerbations in patients with severe asthma
- Anti-histamines- very useful for allergic coughs

Other management options include the following:

- Immunotherapy
  - This involves the injection of pollens or dust mites, but has not been proven to be effective, and may even cause anaphylactic reactions. Hyposensitization is given pre-seasonally (3 weeks prior to onset of season when patient develops asthmatic symptoms), co-seasonal (given just prior to pollen season), and seasonal (given even after the aggravating season is over).
- Alternative therapies
  - Include non-pharmacologic treatment like hypnosis, acupuncture, chiropraxis, breathing control, yoga, etc.

MANAGEMENT OF ASTHMA ACCORDING TO SEVERITY

- Mild Intermittent
  - Short-acting Beta 2 Agonist
- Mild Persistent
  - Short-acting Beta 2 Agonist
  - Low dose of Inhaled Corticosteroids
- Moderate Persistent
  - Short-acting Beta 2 Agonist
  - Low dose of Inhaled Corticosteroids
  - Long-acting Beta 2 Agonist
- Severe Persistent
  - Short-acting Beta 2 Agonist

- o High dose of Inhaled Corticosteroids
- o Long-acting Beta 2 Agonist
- Very Severe Persistent
  - o Short-acting Beta 2 Agonist
  - o High dose of Inhaled Corticosteroids
  - o Long-acting Beta 2 Agonist
  - o Oral Corticosteroids

LIFE-SAVING DEVICES EVERY ASTHMATIC MIUST HAVE

- Asthma inhalers
  - o This device delivers medications straight into the airway, then into the lungs. It relieves symptoms faster, with fewer adverse effects.
- Metered dose inhalers
  - o This device involves a propellant that pushes a metered dose of medication out of the inhaler. Some of these inhalers have indicators that show the remaining dose left.
- Dry powder inhalers
  - o This type of inhaler requires quick breathing; hence, may not be ideal for patients who cannot follow instructions.

USEFUL TIPS FOR ASTHMATICS UNDER MEDICATION

- Record prescriptions and medicines, and save all information about them
- Check the label of your medicines before taking them
- Check the expiration date of each medicine
- Have good compliance to medications as directed by the physician
- Do not share your prescription to other patients
- Inform your physician once symptoms occur after intake of medicine

The above-mentioned treatment options may be traditionally used in the management of asthma; however, some of them pose several side effects, while others have not yet proven to be effective for long-term use.

To serve as alternative, the following are natural remedies to asthma, which are serve as good adjuncts to pharmaceutical treatments.

Figs

Figs are full of nutrients that help in promoting better respiratory health. These nutrients help in draining phlegm (mucus) and in improving breathing.

To use, wash 3 pieces of dried figs. Soak these overnight in 1 cup of water. In the morning, before eating breakfast, eat the figs and drink the soaking water. Make this a daily habit for about 2 months to control asthma symptoms.

Coffee

Caffeine helps in controlling symptoms during an asthma attack by acting as a bronchodilator.

The warmth of the coffee and the caffeine content both work in relaxing and clearing the respiratory tract. These actions help improve breathing.

Stronger coffee (with more caffeine content) tends to provide better results. However, limit daily coffee intake to a maximum of 3 cups of black coffee.

In place of coffee, black tea can be taken. While it is very effective, experts do not recommended using coffee as a regular asthma treatment.

Honey

This is one of the oldest natural treatments for asthma. The alcohol content and the ethereal oils present in honey help in reducing symptoms.

Some people experience relief just by inhaling honey. Adding 1 teaspoon of honey into a cup or glass of hot water is also a good option.

Drink this 3 times per day. To improve sleep and remove phlegm from the throat, mix 1 teaspoon of honey and ½ teaspoon of cinnamon powder. Take this mixture at bedtime.

Lemons

Most people suffering from asthma have low vitamin C levels in the body.

Increasing vitamin C intake, as well as antioxidant intake, helps in decreasing the severity and frequency of asthma symptoms.

Lemon, along with other citrus fruits, is high in vitamin C.

Other great sources include strawberry, blueberry and papaya.

Drink the juice of half a lemon (added to a glass of water) daily to decrease the frequency of attacks.

It is discouraged to drink bottled lemon juice and other similar kinds of drinks.

These may contain additives, colorants and preservatives that may trigger attacks. Also, avoid eating any kind of citrus fruit during an attack because this may worsen the symptoms.

Carom seeds

These are also known as ajwain and Bishop's weed. Carom seeds are effective in treating milder forms of asthma.

The compounds in carom seeds produce bronchodilating effects. This widens the bronchial tree within the lung structure, making it easier to breathe.

Inhaling the steam from boiled water with a teaspoon of the seeds is effective in improving breathing during asthma attacks.

This same mixture can be taken for symptom relief. As topical remedy, the seeds are heated in a pan and wrapped in cotton cloth. Place the cloth with the seeds over the neck and chest area to reduce breathing difficulties.

A paste made from carom seeds is just as effective. The seeds are ground until a paste is formed, then jiggery is added to enhance the benefits.

Eat 1-2 teaspoons of the paste 2 times each day until relief is achieved. The paste is not recommended for people who are also suffering from diabetes.

Omega-3 fatty acids

These are among the healthiest fats that should be included in the diet. Omega-3 fats act similar to leukotriene inhibitors, a class of asthma medication.

These fatty acids prevent the body from producing and releasing leukotrienes.

These are chemicals released by the immune system that causes the airways to become inflamed. Omega-3 fatty acids are naturally obtained from cold water fishes like salmon.

It is also available in supplement form.

When taking supplements, the recommended daily intake is 6 capsules containing 1,000 milligrams of the compound, taken in divided doses throughout the day.

Magnesium

Magnesium is known to promote relaxation of the smooth muscles within the airways.

It can be taken naturally from certain foods, such as green leafy vegetables. It is also available as supplements.

The recommended daily magnesium intake is 600 milligrams.

OTHER DIETARY TIPS

Aside from the aforementioned remedies that help relieve asthma symptoms, healthy eating habits can also improve the condition.

A healthy and well-balanced diet strengthens the body. This helps in better regulation of the immune system and in the suppression of the symptoms.

Eating at least 2 servings of fish every week provides a lot of healthy benefits.

More benefits can be obtained when eating cold-water fish, which are rich in omega-3 fatty acids. Examples of these are salmon (wild caught), mackerel, tuna, herring and cod.

Fresh fruit and vegetables are rich in various nutrients that help strengthen the body, especially the lungs.

Nutrients, such as vitamins C and E, selenium, magnesium and beta-carotene, aid in strengthening and improving lung function.

Whole milk and other dairy products help in reducing asthma symptoms.

However, people who suffer from milk allergies or have lactose intolerance are advised to avoid these foods. These may trigger or worsen asthma.

WHAT TO AVOID

Asthmatic patients suffering from monosodium glutamate (MSG) sensitivity experience flushing and generalized tingling after eating food with MSG.

In addition, studies in Japan have shown that half of the asthmatic patients experience wheezing after alcohol consumption.

Aside from the food mentioned above, asthmatic patients should also avoid cockroach-infested dwellings as children living in these areas become more prone to asthma attacks, especially during summer.

SOME USEFUL DEVICES THAT CAN BE USED AT HOME

- Air Purifiers
  - o Utilizes High Efficiency Particulate Air (HEPA) filters, which can remove particles as small as 3 microns. Although expensive, these devices are said to be 99% efficient.
- Dehumidifiers
  - o Acts by removing water vapor or moisture from the surrounding air. As a result, there is reduction in the growth of dust mites and molds.
- Air conditioners
  - o Also acts as dehumidifier, hence indirectly reducing dust mites. However, regular cleaning should be done to avoid build-up of pollens and dust mites.
- Nebulizers
  - o A device that administers medication in the form of liquid mist. This is usually the preferred device for patients who cannot use inhalers properly, like children.

SPECIAL POPULATION

As mentioned earlier, the goal in the treatment of asthma is basically just to limit inflammation. However, for the following population, treatment may involve additional investigation and additional therapy.

- Asthmatic Patients sensitive to aspirin
  - o Aspirin-sensitive asthma occurs in around 1 to 5% of asthmatic patients. In these patients, asthma attacks become worse with aspirin and other cox-inhibitor intake.
- Elderly asthmatic patients

- o Elderly-onset asthma may occur in some patients. The management for these patients is essentially the same, but more side effects from the medications must be anticipated. Co-morbidities like chronic obstructive pulmonary disease (COPD) at this age group are common.
- Pregnant asthmatic patients
  - o Good control of asthma is required from pregnant women since the condition may affect fetal development. Studies have shown that approximately 1/3 of asthmatic patients improve throughout pregnancy, another 1/3 deteriorate and the other 1/3 remain unchanged.
- Asthmatic cigarette smokers
  - o 20% of asthmatic patients are smokers. Asthmatic smokers are known to have more severe conditions, are admitted more frequently, have faster decline in lung function and are more likely to suffer mortality than non-smokers. In addition, smoking also interferes with the anti-inflammatory actions of corticosteroids. Definitely, smoking cessation leads to significant improvement in the status of the patients.
- Asthmatic patients undergoing surgery
  - o General anesthesia and intubation are not contraindicated to patients with well-controlled asthma. However, surgery may not ensue if the patient is under high doses of corticosteroids as this may delay wound healing.
- Asthmatic patients with Bronchopulmonary Aspergillosis
  - o Although uncommon, this condition results to the inhalation of spores from the species *Aspergillus*. Treatment with antifungal medications may be required to prevent exacerbations of asthma.

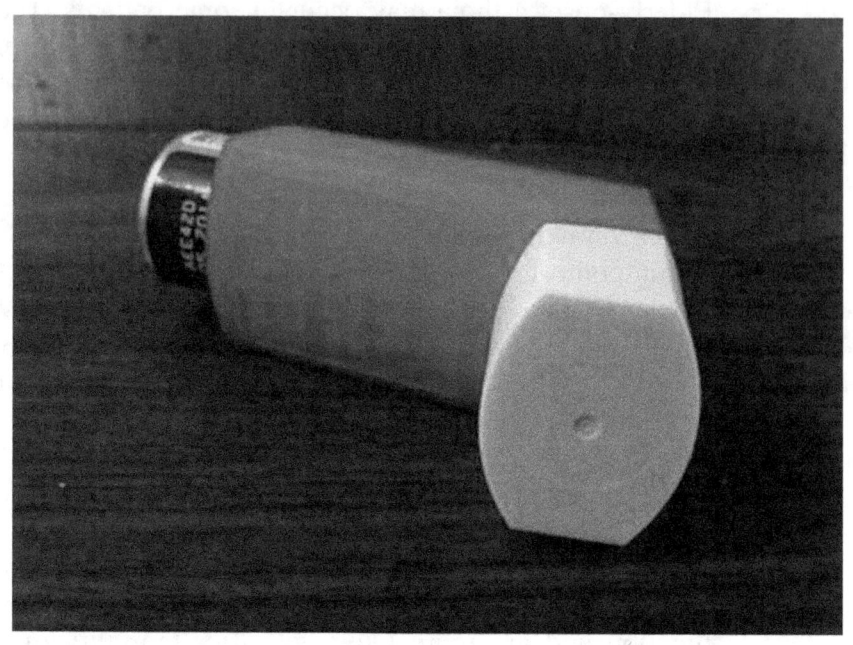

Relying on medication isn't always necessary

(Image Credit – ParentingPatch
http://commons.wikimedia.org/wiki/File:Asthma_Medication_Inhaler.JPG)

CHAPTER 4
Herbs to Relieve Asthma Symptoms

Herbs are just as effective as asthma medication and certain foods in relieving and treating symptoms.

Ginger

This is one of the most popular, commonly used natural remedies for a wide range of illnesses. Ginger can also help in the treatment of asthma.

As discovered through scientific studies, ginger contains active compounds that effectively reduce inflammation in the airways and inhibit contractions of the muscles that line the respiratory tract.

These effects help in alleviating breathing difficulties during asthma attacks. A few studies have also found that taking ginger with certain asthma medications enhances relaxant effects on the muscles.

There are several ways of using ginger. Common preparations include the following:

- Mix equal portions of ginger juice (freshly squeezed), honey, and pomegranate juice. Take 1 tablespoon of this mixture 2-3 times each day.
- Another way to take ginger is to have it ground or mashed. Mix 1 teaspoon of it to half a cup of water. Drink 1 tablespoon of this mixture before going to bed at night.
- Get a 1-inch piece of ginger. Slice into smaller pieces. Boil water in a small pot. Add the slices of ginger. Turn off the heat and allow the ginger to steep in water for about 5 minutes. Cool before drinking.

- Taking a decoction made with ginger and fenugreek is one effective way of detoxifying the lungs. To prepare, boil a cup of water and a tablespoon of fenugreek seeds. Add 1 tablespoon of ginger juice and a tablespoon of honey. Drink this in the morning as well as in the evening.
- The simplest way to take ginger is by slicing raw ginger root and eating it with salt.

Garlic

Garlic can treat several ailments, including asthma. It is one of the herbs with a very long history of medicinal use.

Garlic helps in clearing up congestion within the lungs, which actually occurs during the early stages of an asthma attack.

To use during an asthma attack, combine ¼ cup of milk and 2-3 pieces of cloves in a small pot. Bring to a boil. Remove from heat and set aside to cool down to room temperature. Drink.

Onions

Onions are rich in compounds that act as anti-inflammatory agents in the body. These compounds reduce the constriction within the airways that occur during an asthma attack.

The sulfur content of onion is effective in reducing any inflammation in the lungs.

Eating raw onion is enough to clear the airways for improved breathing. Eating cooked onion is also fine, especially if raw onion is not an option flavor-wise.

Mustard Oil

Mustard oil can help in reducing symptoms during an asthma attack. It clears the airways and helps in restoring normal respiration pattern.

To use, place a small amount of mustard oil in a small pot and add a few drops of camphor. Heat this mixture over low fire.

Remove and transfer the oil mixture into a small bowl.

Allow to cool slightly, or until it's comfortably warm. Gently apply over the upper back and chest areas. Massage.

Perform this several times until asthma symptoms subside.

Eucalyptus Oil

Pure oil extracted from eucalyptus has very effective decongestant properties. As discovered by experts, this oil contains eucalyptol.

This chemical effectively breaks up mucus, in turn relieving congestion within the lungs.

To use, apply a small amount of eucalyptus oil on a clean paper towel. Place it by the head, over the pillow so that the aroma can be breathed in while sleeping.

The oil can also be added to steam inhalation treatment. Boil a pot of water and add 2-3 drops of eucalyptus oil.

Place the face over the steam and inhale deeply for relief.

Evening Primrose Oil

This oil contains abundant amounts of GLA, one type of essential fatty acid.

The body converts GLA into a compound that acts as an anti-inflammatory agent. Evening primrose oil is available in supplement capsules.

The recommended dose is 2 capsules (500mg each) taken 3 times per day. This may cause mild stomach upset in some individuals. To prevent this, take evening primrose oil with meals.

Quercetin

This is a bioflavonoid that prevents the body from releasing histamine that causes asthma symptoms.

Quercetin is available in supplement form.

The recommended daily dose is at 500 milligrams, taken 3 times per day. The best time to take this supplement is 20 minutes before eating a meal.

Turmeric

This is a spice commonly used in Indian cooking. It is a yellow-colored spice that is also used in treating various illnesses.

It is a top anti-inflammatory food that can help in alleviating asthma symptoms. In the body, compounds in turmeric suppress the release of COX-2 prostaglandins.

These are compounds that resemble hormones and are involved in the inflammatory cascade.

To use turmeric for asthma relief, mix 1 teaspoon of the spice to 1 cup of warm milk. Drink 3 times per day.

Turmeric is also available in supplement form, either as capsules or tinctures.

Ma Huang

This herb is more popularly known as ephedra.

In the body, ma huang produces a bronchodilating effect, effectively opening up constricted air passages. This herb is only to be taken under medical supervision.

It can increase heart rate and irritability, which may turn fatal if there are underlying disorders such as heart ailments.

Reishi mushrooms

These are most popularly used in Chinese traditional medicine.

These contain a lot of chemicals that have very strong immune-building and anti-inflammatory actions.

It also helps in strengthening the lungs and improving its function. Reishi mushrooms are available whole, fresh, or dried. They're also available in tincture form.

CHAPTER 5
Preventing Asthma

Prevention is the key to successful asthma management. By identifying the triggers and avoiding them, it's definitely possible to live a symptom-free life.

Avoiding triggers

Triggers are abundantly found in the environment. By identifying specific triggers, elimination and avoidance is easier. The most common triggers are dust, molds, pollen, and pet dander. Here are a few tips to avoiding these:

- Air conditioners can help in preventing pollen and dust from getting inside the home. These appliances are most helpful during pollen season. These also help in keeping indoor humidity low, which helps in reducing asthma symptoms and improving breathing. Using an air conditioner also helps in reducing the exposure to dust mites.
- Do not smoke. Also, avoid areas frequented by smokers to avoid exposure to secondhand smoke. Smoke from cigarettes irritates the air passages, which in turn can trigger or worsen symptoms of asthma.
- Avoid huddling in front of wood-burning stove, open campfire, or fireplaces. The smoke from the burning wood may trigger or worsen symptoms.
- If asthma is triggered by cold, dry air, cover the mouth and nose with a scarf when going out in cold weather.
- Decontaminating home décor helps in reducing triggers inside the house. Removing dust and discouraging dust

accumulation is one major way of controlling asthma and its symptoms. Use dustproof covers on mattresses, pillows, etc.

- Maintaining optimal humidity helps in controlling asthma triggered by environmental temperatures. Using dehumidifiers may be necessary for those who live in damp climates. Humidifiers may be necessary inside the home when living in dry climates.
- Prevent mold growth. There are several ways to reduce or discourage mold growth, such as regular cleaning of damp areas like bathrooms and kitchen sinks. Also, remove damp firewood and moldy leaves in the yard to prevent spores from getting released into the air.
- Not having pets in the house is the best way of preventing exposure to dander. If that's not an option, have the pets stay in specific areas – away from rooms frequented by family members who suffer from asthma. Pets should be regularly groomed and bathed to reduce dander in the surroundings.

Boost the body's health and immunity

Keeping asthma under control also requires keeping the rest of the body healthy. Improved immunity also helps in reducing the frequency and severity of symptoms.

Better overall health helps in strengthening and improving the functions of the various organs, including the lungs.

Some things that help keep the body healthy include:

- Regular exercise
- Maintaining healthy weight
- Healthy, balanced, nutritious diet

Controlling GERD and heartburn

Studies have found a link between heartburn and GERD (gastroesophageal reflux disease) and asthma.

Acid reflux in these health conditions may reduce lung function and damage the respiratory passages. Treatments for GERD have been found to also reduce asthma symptoms.

Another way to control GERD and improve asthma symptoms is to adjust meal times.

Eat smaller and more frequent meals throughout the day, instead of 3 big meals. Before going to bed, avoid eating anything.

Lying down after a meal causes stomach acids to rise into the esophagus and cause heartburn.

LONG TERM PREVENTION AND CONTROL

For long-term management, control, and prevention of symptoms, simply follow these tips:

- Reduce daily protein intake to about 10% of the recommended daily caloric needs. Also, take most of the body's protein needs from plant sources such as beans. Proteins play an important role in the development of asthma symptoms, as these may carry triggers.
- Substitute milk and dairy products with other calcium sources. There is still ongoing debate on whether milk helps in asthma treatment or if it is a trigger for asthma. As has been mentioned earlier, people who have milk allergies or with lactose intolerance should avoid these foods. Also, if asthma symptoms tend to worsen with these foods, eliminate them from the diet. Choose other calcium sources such as kale and spinach.
- Eat organic vegetables, fruits, and meat products such as organic chicken and grass-fed beef. Organic food and food products have less artificial chemicals that can reduce lung function, act as asthma triggers, and cause health to deteriorate.
- Drink lots of water, at least 8 glasses, in a day. Increase water intake on humid or dry days, after exercising or sweating a lot. Water helps in keeping a healthy balance in

the body. It also helps in thinning mucus accumulation in the lungs, making it easier to expectorate.

- Avoid processed foods and those with additives. These are possible sources of triggers. Also, some of the chemicals in these foods negatively affect health, making a person more susceptible to health problems like asthma. Reduce the intake of anything that contains bad carbohydrates, such as heavily processed forms of starch and sugar, partially hydrogenated and hydrogenated fats, flavorings, sweeteners, and artificial additives.

- Avoid foods that contain sulfites and nitrites/nitrates. Most people who suffer from asthma are also sensitive to sulfites, nitrites and/or nitrates. These are often found in processed and preserved meats such as hotdogs, deli meats and bacon. These are also found in wine, beers and cheeses. People who are sensitive to sulfites may benefit from taking vitamin B12 and molybdenum. These aid in metabolizing and oxidizing sulfites, which reduces the risk of triggering an asthma attack.

- Engage in regular daily exercise. Include a good balance of resistance training, stretching (such as yoga) and aerobic exercise. Avoid performing any exercise in dry and cold air, as doing so can trigger an asthma attack. Also, remember to warm up first with some low-intensity routines for at least 10 minutes.

- Include antioxidants in daily health regimen. These are available in natural foods like fruits. These are also available in supplements. Antioxidants reduce free radicals in the body. Free radicals worsen inflammation. By reducing and inhibiting these substances, inflammation and associated asthma symptoms are effectively reduced. Good antioxidants to take daily include vitamins E, A and C, bioflavonoids (e.g., rutin, hesperidin), bromelain, NAC (N-acetyl cysteine), and quercetin. Bromelain, in particular, is a pineapple enzyme that has very potent anti-inflammatory action, especially when taken on an empty stomach.

- Keep your house clean and make your environment conducive for your health. Wash your linens weekly in hot water and sundry them. As much as possible, beddings should be made with synthetic or cotton material.

- Monitor lung function regularly. It is important to note that two to three days before an attack, lung function decreases. A 20% decrease in the peak flow meter indicates an incoming asthma attack.

BONUS CHAPTER
Asthma Myths vs. Facts

MYTH: An individual allergic to a certain allergen can no longer be allergic to another.

FACT: An individual allergic to a certain kind of allergen can still be allergic to another, since cross-reactions among particles can occur. Hence, hyposensitization against different kinds of allergens must still be done.

MYTH: Allergies do not require immediate attention or medications

FACT: A lot of people suffer from allergic conditions, which lead to lost time from school and work. Severe forms of allergy, as in the case of anaphylactic reactions may even lead to death.

MYTH: Each patient suffers from the same severity and intensity of asthma

FACT: Severity and intensity of asthma varies among patients. Hence, treatment must also be tailored according to the needs of the patient.

MYTH: Asthma medications are unsafe because they contain steroids

FACT: Asthmatic patients usually utilize inhaled steroids; hence they do not result to systemic side effects. In addition, steroids are essential in the reduction and control of attacks.

MYTH: Asthmatic patients cannot engage in sports

FACT: Patients with asthma can still engage themselves in sports activities for as long as their condition is well controlled, and that they are aware of what to do in case an attack occurs.

MYTH: Adults cannot suffer from allergies

FACT: Allergic reactions to food and medicines can happen to everyone from all ages. Some cases of asthma can occur during adulthood and even during elderly years.

MYTH: The lungs will eventually improve with medications and may become immune to asthma attacks

FACT: Asthma is an incurable condition. However, it can be controlled and its symptoms can be managed. Hence, continuous medication is needed.

MYTH: Asthmatic children become cured after tonsillectomy (removal of tonsils)

FACT: Enlarged tonsils are only a precipitating factor that leads to asthma, but it does not resolve the fact that the child is allergic to a substance, and this still needs to be addressed.

BONUS CHAPTER
Famous People with Asthma

- John F. Kennedy
  - He was the 35th president of the United States until his assassination in 1963. He was diagnosed with Asthma, among many other diseases, and yet, he was still able to enjoy playing sports with his family.
- Ludwig von Beethoven
  - He was a famous German composer and pianist. In 1796, he began to have hearing problems. After he suffered an attack, he used to go to the country and take a sketchbook with him.
- Elizabeth Taylor
  - Both talented and beautiful, she was known as one of Hollywood's most talented actresses.
- Theodore Roosevelt
  - He was the 26th president of the United States. Aside from asthma, he also suffered from poor eyesight and epileptic seizure

SOURCES:

- Longo, et al. (2012). Harrison's Principles of Internal Medicine. New York, NY: McGraw-Hill Companies
- Arora, A. (2012). 5 Steps to Combat Asthma and Allergies. New Delhi, India: Sterling Publishers (P) Ltd.
- Famous People with Asthma. (2008, January 17). Retrieved from http://www.disabled-world.com/artman/publish/asthma-famous.shtml
- History of Asthma. Retrieved from http://www.allergyandasthma.com/home/articles/history-of-asthma

Conclusion

Thank you again for downloading this book!

I hope this book was able to help you understand what asthma is and how symptoms could be effectively managed and controlled.

This condition may often prevent sufferers from living a full life because of the precautions they have to take.

But, with a proper management plan and with the right preventive measures, as well as a healthy diet and supplementation, you can still enjoy life to the fullest.

The next step is to start eating healthier food, avoiding all known asthma triggers like additives and sulfites.

Furthermore, tell others about this book so they, too, can live a full life that is asthma-free.

Finally, if you enjoyed this book, then I'd like to ask you for a favor, would you be kind enough to leave a review for this book on Amazon?

It'd be greatly appreciated!

Please leave a review for this book on Amazon!

Thank you and good luck!

www.ingramcontent.com/pod-product-compliance
Lightning Source LLC
Chambersburg PA
CBHW070450290526
45791CB00005B/2111